This book belongs to

_____

My Goals

My weight goal: _____

Nutrition strategies to reach my weight goal:

_____

_____

_____

_____

_____

Daily activity goals:

_____

_____

_____

Notes:

My Progress

Date	Weight	Waist	Hip

Date:

How many hours did I sleep last night?

How am I feeling?

What is my stress level?
(1= very relax, 8 = very stressed)

1   2   3   4   5   6   7   8

Today, I will …

Date:

Time	Food & Drinks	Amount

Time	Activity	Minutes

Date:

How many hours did I sleep last night?

How am I feeling?

What is my stress level?
(1= very relax, 8 = very stressed)

1   2   3   4   5   6   7   8

Today, I will …

Date:

Time	Food & Drinks	Amount

Time	Activity	Minutes

Date:

How many hours did I sleep last night?

How am I feeling?

What is my stress level?
(1= very relax, 8 = very stressed)

1   2   3   4   5   6   7   8

Today, I will …

Date:

Time	Food & Drinks	Amount

Time	Activity	Minutes

Date:

How many hours did I sleep last night?

How am I feeling?

What is my stress level?
(1= very relax, 8 = very stressed)

| 1 | 2 | 3 | 4 | 5 | 6 | 7 | 8 |

Today, I will …

Date:

Time	Food & Drinks	Amount

Time	Activity	Minutes

Date:

How many hours did I sleep last night?

How am I feeling?

What is my stress level?
(1= very relax, 8 = very stressed)

1   2   3   4   5   6   7   8

Today, I will …

Date:

Time	Food & Drinks	Amount

Time	Activity	Minutes

Date:

How many hours did I sleep last night?

How am I feeling?

What is my stress level?
(1= very relax, 8 = very stressed)

1   2   3   4   5   6   7   8

Today, I will …

Date:

Time	Food & Drinks	Amount

Time	Activity	Minutes

17

Date:

How many hours did I sleep last night?

How am I feeling?

What is my stress level?
(1= very relax, 8 = very stressed)

1   2   3   4   5   6   7   8

Today, I will …

Date:

Time	Food & Drinks	Amount

Time	Activity	Minutes

Date:

How many hours did I sleep last night?

How am I feeling?

What is my stress level?
(1= very relax, 8 = very stressed)

1   2   3   4   5   6   7   8

Today, I will …

Date:

Time	Food & Drinks	Amount

Time	Activity	Minutes

Date:

How many hours did I sleep last night?

```
┌─────────────────────────────────┐
│                                 │
│                                 │
└─────────────────────────────────┘
```

How am I feeling?

What is my stress level?
(1= very relax, 8 = very stressed)

1   2   3   4   5   6   7   8

Today, I will …

Date:

Time	Food & Drinks	Amount

Time	Activity	Minutes

Date:

How many hours did I sleep last night?

How am I feeling?

What is my stress level?
(1= very relax, 8 = very stressed)

1	2	3	4	5	6	7	8

Today, I will …

Date:

Time	Food & Drinks	Amount

Time	Activity	Minutes

Date:

How many hours did I sleep last night?

How am I feeling?

What is my stress level?
(1= very relax, 8 = very stressed)

1   2   3   4   5   6   7   8

Today, I will …

Date:

Time	Food & Drinks	Amount

Time	Activity	Minutes

Date:

How many hours did I sleep last night?

How am I feeling?

What is my stress level?
(1= very relax, 8 = very stressed)

1   2   3   4   5   6   7   8

Today, I will …

Date:

Time	Food & Drinks	Amount

Time	Activity	Minutes

Date:

How many hours did I sleep last night?

How am I feeling?

What is my stress level?
(1= very relax, 8 = very stressed)

1   2   3   4   5   6   7   8

Today, I will …

Date:

Time	Food & Drinks	Amount

Time	Activity	Minutes

Date:

How many hours did I sleep last night?

How am I feeling?

What is my stress level?
(1= very relax, 8 = very stressed)

1   2   3   4   5   6   7   8

Today, I will …

Date:

Time	Food & Drinks	Amount

Time	Activity	Minutes

Date:

How many hours did I sleep last night?

How am I feeling?

What is my stress level?
(1= very relax, 8 = very stressed)

1   2   3   4   5   6   7   8

Today, I will …

Date:

Time	Food & Drinks	Amount

Time	Activity	Minutes

Date:

How many hours did I sleep last night?

How am I feeling?

What is my stress level?
(1= very relax, 8 = very stressed)

1   2   3   4   5   6   7   8

Today, I will …

Date:

Time	Food & Drinks	Amount

Time	Activity	Minutes

Date:

How many hours did I sleep last night?

How am I feeling?

What is my stress level?
(1= very relax, 8 = very stressed)

1   2   3   4   5   6   7   8

Today, I will …

Date:

Time	Food & Drinks	Amount

Time	Activity	Minutes

Date:

How many hours did I sleep last night?

```
┌─────────────────────────────────────┐
│                                     │
│                                     │
└─────────────────────────────────────┘
```

How am I feeling?

What is my stress level?
(1= very relax, 8 = very stressed)

1   2   3   4   5   6   7   8

Today, I will …

Date:

Time	Food & Drinks	Amount

Time	Activity	Minutes

Date:

How many hours did I sleep last night?

How am I feeling?

What is my stress level?
(1= very relax, 8 = very stressed)

1   2   3   4   5   6   7   8

Today, I will …

Date:

Time	Food & Drinks	Amount

Time	Activity	Minutes

Date:

How many hours did I sleep last night?

How am I feeling?

What is my stress level?
(1= very relax, 8 = very stressed)

1   2   3   4   5   6   7   8

Today, I will …

Date:

Time	Food & Drinks	Amount

Time	Activity	Minutes

Date:

How many hours did I sleep last night?

How am I feeling?

What is my stress level?
(1= very relax, 8 = very stressed)

1   2   3   4   5   6   7   8

Today, I will …

Date:

Time	Food & Drinks	Amount

Time	Activity	Minutes

Date:

How many hours did I sleep last night?

How am I feeling?

What is my stress level?
(1= very relax, 8 = very stressed)

1   2   3   4   5   6   7   8

Today, I will …

Date:

Time	Food & Drinks	Amount

Time	Activity	Minutes

Date:

How many hours did I sleep last night?

How am I feeling?

What is my stress level?
(1 = very relax, 8 = very stressed)

1   2   3   4   5   6   7   8

Today, I will …

Date:

Time	Food & Drinks	Amount

Time	Activity	Minutes

Date:

How many hours did I sleep last night?

How am I feeling?

What is my stress level?
(1= very relax, 8 = very stressed)

1   2   3   4   5   6   7   8

Today, I will …

Date:

Time	Food & Drinks	Amount

Time	Activity	Minutes

Date:

How many hours did I sleep last night?

How am I feeling?

What is my stress level?
(1= very relax, 8 = very stressed)

1   2   3   4   5   6   7   8

Today, I will …

Date:

Time	Food & Drinks	Amount

Time	Activity	Minutes

Date:

How many hours did I sleep last night?

How am I feeling?

What is my stress level?
(1= very relax, 8 = very stressed)

1   2   3   4   5   6   7   8

Today, I will ...

Date:

Time	Food & Drinks	Amount

Time	Activity	Minutes

Date:

How many hours did I sleep last night?

How am I feeling?

What is my stress level?
(1= very relax, 8 = very stressed)

1   2   3   4   5   6   7   8

Today, I will …

Date:

Time	Food & Drinks	Amount

Time	Activity	Minutes

Date:

How many hours did I sleep last night?

┌─────────────────────────────────┐
│   │
│   │
└─────────────────────────────────┘

How am I feeling?

What is my stress level?
(1= very relax, 8 = very stressed)

1   2   3   4   5   6   7   8

Today, I will …

Date:

Time	Food & Drinks	Amount

Time	Activity	Minutes

Date:

How many hours did I sleep last night?

How am I feeling?

What is my stress level?
(1= very relax, 8 = very stressed)

1   2   3   4   5   6   7   8

Today, I will …

Date:

Time	Food & Drinks	Amount

Time	Activity	Minutes

Date:

How many hours did I sleep last night?

How am I feeling?

What is my stress level?
(1= very relax, 8 = very stressed)

1   2   3   4   5   6   7   8

Today, I will …

Date:

Time	Food & Drinks	Amount

Time	Activity	Minutes

Date:

How many hours did I sleep last night?

How am I feeling?

What is my stress level?
(1= very relax, 8 = very stressed)

1   2   3   4   5   6   7   8

Today, I will ...

Date:

Time	Food & Drinks	Amount

Time	Activity	Minutes

Date:

How many hours did I sleep last night?

How am I feeling?

What is my stress level?
(1= very relax, 8 = very stressed)

1   2   3   4   5   6   7   8

Today, I will …

Date:

Time	Food & Drinks	Amount

Time	Activity	Minutes

Date:

How many hours did I sleep last night?

How am I feeling?

What is my stress level?
(1= very relax, 8 = very stressed)

1   2   3   4   5   6   7   8

Today, I will …

Date:

Time	Food & Drinks	Amount

Time	Activity	Minutes

Date:

How many hours did I sleep last night?

```
┌─────────────────────────────────┐
│                                 │
│                                 │
└─────────────────────────────────┘
```

How am I feeling?

What is my stress level?
(1= very relax, 8 = very stressed)

1   2   3   4   5   6   7   8

Today, I will ...

Date:

Time	Food & Drinks	Amount

Time	Activity	Minutes

Date:

How many hours did I sleep last night?

How am I feeling?

What is my stress level?
(1= very relax, 8 = very stressed)

1   2   3   4   5   6   7   8

Today, I will ...

Date:

Time	Food & Drinks	Amount

Time	Activity	Minutes

Date:

How many hours did I sleep last night?

How am I feeling?

What is my stress level?
(1= very relax, 8 = very stressed)

1   2   3   4   5   6   7   8

Today, I will …

Date:

Time	Food & Drinks	Amount

Time	Activity	Minutes

Date:

How many hours did I sleep last night?

How am I feeling?

What is my stress level?
(1= very relax, 8 = very stressed)

1   2   3   4   5   6   7   8

Today, I will …

Date:

Time	Food & Drinks	Amount

Time	Activity	Minutes

Date:

How many hours did I sleep last night?

How am I feeling?

What is my stress level?
(1= very relax, 8 = very stressed)

1   2   3   4   5   6   7   8

Today, I will ...

Date:

Time	Food & Drinks	Amount

Time	Activity	Minutes

Date:

How many hours did I sleep last night?

How am I feeling?

What is my stress level?
(1= very relax, 8 = very stressed)

1   2   3   4   5   6   7   8

Today, I will …

Date:

Time	Food & Drinks	Amount

Time	Activity	Minutes

Date:

How many hours did I sleep last night?

| |
| |

How am I feeling?

What is my stress level?
(1= very relax, 8 = very stressed)

1   2   3   4   5   6   7   8

Today, I will …

Date:

Time	Food & Drinks	Amount

Time	Activity	Minutes

Date:

How many hours did I sleep last night?

How am I feeling?

What is my stress level?
(1= very relax, 8 = very stressed)

1   2   3   4   5   6   7   8

Today, I will ...

Date:

Time	Food & Drinks	Amount

Time	Activity	Minutes

Date:

How many hours did I sleep last night?

How am I feeling?

What is my stress level?
(1= very relax, 8 = very stressed)

1   2   3   4   5   6   7   8

Today, I will …

Date:

Time	Food & Drinks	Amount

Time	Activity	Minutes

Date:

How many hours did I sleep last night?

How am I feeling?

What is my stress level?
(1= very relax, 8 = very stressed)

1   2   3   4   5   6   7   8

Today, I will …

Date:

Time	Food & Drinks	Amount

Time	Activity	Minutes

Date:

How many hours did I sleep last night?

How am I feeling?

What is my stress level?
(1= very relax, 8 = very stressed)

1   2   3   4   5   6   7   8

Today, I will …

Date:

Time	Food & Drinks	Amount

Time	Activity	Minutes

Date:

How many hours did I sleep last night?

How am I feeling?

What is my stress level?
(1= very relax, 8 = very stressed)

1   2   3   4   5   6   7   8

Today, I will ...

Date:

Time	Food & Drinks	Amount

Time	Activity	Minutes

Date:

How many hours did I sleep last night?

How am I feeling?

What is my stress level?
(1= very relax, 8 = very stressed)

1   2   3   4   5   6   7   8

Today, I will …

Date:

Time	Food & Drinks	Amount

Time	Activity	Minutes

Date:

How many hours did I sleep last night?

How am I feeling?

What is my stress level?
(1= very relax, 8 = very stressed)

1   2   3   4   5   6   7   8

Today, I will ...

Date:

Time	Food & Drinks	Amount

Time	Activity	Minutes

Date:

How many hours did I sleep last night?

How am I feeling?

What is my stress level?
(1= very relax, 8 = very stressed)

1   2   3   4   5   6   7   8

Today, I will ...

Date:

Time	Food & Drinks	Amount

Time	Activity	Minutes

Date:

How many hours did I sleep last night?

How am I feeling?

What is my stress level?
(1= very relax, 8 = very stressed)

1   2   3   4   5   6   7   8

Today, I will …

Date:

Time	Food & Drinks	Amount

Time	Activity	Minutes

Date:

How many hours did I sleep last night?

How am I feeling?

What is my stress level?
(1= very relax, 8 = very stressed)

1   2   3   4   5   6   7   8

Today, I will …

Date:

Time	Food & Drinks	Amount

Time	Activity	Minutes

UNIT OF MEASUREMENT

1 teaspoon = 5 milliliters

3 teaspoons = 1 tablespoon

1 tablespoon = 3 teaspoons

1 tablespoon = 15 milliliters

1 fluid ounce = 2 tablespoons

1 cup = 8 fluid ounces

1 cup = 16 tablespoons

1 pint = 2 cups

1 quart = 2 pints

1 quart = 4 cups

1 gallon = 4 quarts

1 gallon = 8 pints

1 gallon = 3.4 liters

1 pound = 16 ounces

1 kilogram = 2.2 pounds